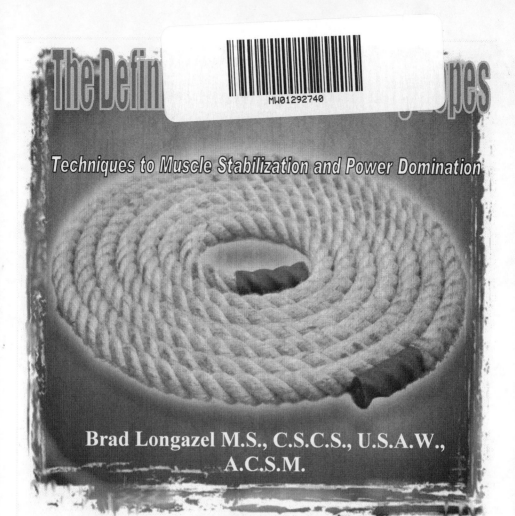

The Definitive Guide to Battling Ropes

Techniques to Muscle Stabilization and Power Domination

Brad Longazel M.S., C.S.C.S., U.S.A.W., A.C.S.M.

1

Copyright © 2012 by Brad Longazel
All Rights Reserved

For more information please visit

www.cpifitness.com

www.definitiveropes.com

Disclaimer

The information in this book is offered for educational purposes only; the reader is cautioned that there is an inherent risk assumed by anyone who engages in any form of physical activity. With that in mind, readers who choose to participate in this strength and conditioning program should check with their physician prior to initiating such activities. Anyone participating in these activities should understand that such training initiatives may be dangerous if performed incorrectly. The author assumes no liability for injury; this manual is purely an educational guide designed for those who are already proficient with the demands of such exercise programming and physical activity.

Table of Contents

Section 1: Introduction

The Beauty of Battling Ropes

This manual illustrates how the unique and multi-faceted benefits of battling-rope exercises add dimensions to physical training that are difficult to achieve through other, more traditional training tools.

The popularity of battling ropes has tremendously increased in recent years. Their popularity stems from the both fact that they have distinct advantages over most other training tools and the fact that people of all athletic backgrounds and abilities - from Olympic athletes and MMA fighters to weight-loss hopefuls can benefit from training with battling ropes.

Battling-rope training is an inherently non-impact, versatile exercise system that can be used for rehabilitation purposes as well as for power development by elite-level athletes. At the same time that they are non-impact exercises, they also provide a taxing and effective workout – a rare combination that makes battling ropes an ideal training exercise. Additionally, because the exercises are

6

non-impact, risk of injury is minimal as compared to the use of traditional free weights.

Moreover, battling ropes provide instant performance feedback that is not possible with traditional weights. Traditional weight-training involves increasing weights in order to increase difficulty and promote greater gains, but the weights can only be increased in set increments. As a result, there is no real-time means by which to gauge force/speed production. By contrast, battling ropes' difficulty is created instantaneously and the feedback as to force/speed production is immediate. The larger and faster the waves are in the movement, the more difficult the movement is and therefore the greater the force produced. Prime movers such as the shoulders, lats, and quadriceps naturally respond by working to create force.

There are very few training tools that have this distinct advantage and that don't cost a small fortune. So find a rope, anchor it to a solid surface and take advantage of an amazing workout.

7

Intrinsic Muscle Action

The real beauty and unique benefit of using battling ropes is the strength you will gain in the small intrinsic muscles of your body. Using battling ropes causes all of the small muscles of your body turn on by moving the ropes faster which increases the production of force and speed. The affected muscles include the core stabilizers in your torso and rotator cuff muscles in your shoulders. Those muscle groups are vital to a healthy and functional body.

Frequently, exercise and development of those muscle groups go unaddressed by traditional weight training programs. Using battling ropes almost guarantees they will be worked. Each time you move your arm or arms further away from your body with a weight in your hands, a tremendous amount of stress is placed on your shoulders. Compensating for the off balance load in front of your body core stabilizers are turned on to balance and keep the body upright. Multiple movements in this guide require extended

8

arms and intrinsic muscle action is found. Dynamic stabilization from the core creates a strong body that is capable of creating and transferring power from the upper body to the lower body and vice versa.

Power Development

Creating and transferring force, which is the ability to generate power with your body, is the heart of athleticism. Whether it is swinging a baseball bat, throwing a punch, or jumping, the more force you can produce the better you are at these tasks. The unique nature of battling-rope movements helps you to create force in more than just a linear path, which is how traditional weight training programs are commonly designed and which is why battling ropes reaps more of an overall benefit. The rhythmic nature of the waves you create when you move the ropers generates force throughout your body because you will naturally resist the forward momentum, i.e. the pull, of the ropes as well as the force of gravity that simultaneously pulls the ropes down. That

9

resistance requires multiple muscle contractions on both the front and backside of your body as all of the muscles will work to create opposing force and power.

Training the core muscles in this way develops excellent core stabilization. Stabilized core muscles allow any force that stems from the lower body (such as a jump) to be transferred all the way up the body to the arms. For example, when you throw a punch, core stabilization allows all the force from your legs to transfer to your fist, leading to one powerful punch. Power is also important outside of athletics. Have you ever stumbled or gotten a little off balance? Speed and power development increase the rate at which your muscles contract. The more powerful and quicker you are, the better the chances are that you will catch yourself before you hit the ground.

Selecting the Right Rope

Battling ropes come in varied lengths and thicknesses. Selecting a rope that will meet your training needs is not a difficult task. First, consider the amount of space you have available in your training location. Normally a 30' rope should fit most gyms and can also likely be used in most home gyms or driveways. Thirty feet of rope provides enough weight to still be challenging for advanced beginners to intermediate athletes. For stronger, larger athletes, a longer or thicker rope will be necessary.

If your space permits, forty feet is a more ideal length. It is more versatile with respect to all of the possible movements and will provide a degree of resistance that is suited to more seasoned fitness enthusiasts.

Thickness of the rope is important to consider as well. The heavier the rope is the more work that is required to create full waves all the way down to the anchor point. For example, a 40' 1.5in. rope weights 22lbs. while a 40' 2.0 in. rope weighs 33lbs. Thus, the 2.0 in. rope is the more ideal. Again, if your space or budget requires a 30' foot, 1 in. rope, you can still achieve an effective workout so long as you maintain a high intensity level throughout.

11

Anchoring the Rope

One of the most important steps in using battling ropes is selecting an anchor point that can support the weight of both you and the rope. A lot of the unique movements of battling ropes require a sturdy anchor point that can support your weight. Make an appropriate selection before starting to train with ropes. Do's and don'ts for anchor points are set out below:

Great selections

- Support beams that span from floor to ceiling

- Trees

- Floor secured power racks

Okay selection

- Wall mounted anchors

- Loaded weight trees

Do not use

- Weight plates / kettlebells

- Training partners foot / hands

- Any other moveable object

If you do not have an anchor point from one of the great selection locations listed, do not perform any of the exercises that require leaning or pulling on the ropes to support your weight. The potential risk of injury is far too high to outweigh the benefits from this style of training.

Grip Identification

There are two main hand positions: the underhand and overhand grip.

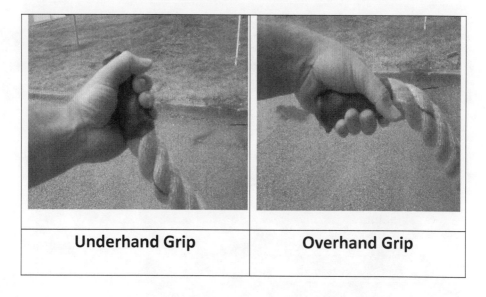

| Underhand Grip | Overhand Grip |

The underhand grip generally places the wrist in a more neutral position. It is used in overhead movements because the neutral positioning of the wrist results in less stress on the shoulder joint, (also referred to as the glenohumeral joint).

The overhand grip is used for movements in which the arms stay at or below shoulder-level. In those movements, using the overhand grip creates a more natural movement of the shoulder joint which again minimizes stress.

Grip selection also impacts muscular activation for most of the movements. For instance, using an underhand grip for overhead movements ensures activation of the shoulder muscles that yields more effective training and better results.

Stance Selections

Depending on your goals, you may choose to either stand or kneel when performing the movements described in this manual.

- **Kneeling**

Kneeling on a pad while moving the ropes prevents use of the lower body muscles for stabilization. This results in concentrating the stabilization work of your muscles up higher and into the core and hips. So if you want to focus on these areas, kneeling is the way to go. Rope work from a kneeling stance is also a great option for individuals with knee or hip discomfort or injuries.

- **Standing**

Standing will force not only your core muscles but also the muscle groups in your lower body to work in order to achieve stabilization. The posterior muscle groups of the glutes and hamstrings will be forced to engage in order to resist the forward pull generated by the momentum of the ropes. Standing will also exercise your core muscles but the stress will be shared by the lower-body muscle groups. For this reason, if your goal is to concentrate on centralized core stabilization, you will want to use the kneeling position. And when you want to concentrate on total body strength, you should use the standing position.

15

Always Keep Neutral Spinal Posture

Use of ropes causes forces to be generated in and transferred from the lower body to the upper body. Accordingly, properly performing the movements and maximizing the benefits hinges on being able to lock down your core while moving the ropes and keeping your spine in a neutral position. Thus, learning what good posture and a neutral spine are and how to maintain them throughout the exercise movements pays huge dividends with respect to developing a solid and stable core.

So what is good spinal posture? There are four areas of the spine that need to be in proper alignment with each movement: the head, shoulders, thoracic spine (upper back), and lumbar spine (lower spine).

- **Head /neck posture**

The ideal head position places the head centered and equally balanced between the shoulders; the back of the head should fall directly in line with the arch of the upper back.

16

- **Shoulder posture**

The position of the shoulders is directly influenced by the scapula. Good shoulder position pulls the scapula back and down which will limit slouching of the upper back. A quick way to assume proper shoulder posture is with the "thumbs up and out" movement. Start with both arms relaxed at your sides. Make the thumbs up hand sign with your thumbs parallel to the floor and rotate your thumbs out away from your body as hard as you can. This will pull your shoulders back. Once your shoulders are pulled back relax your arms without relaxing your back and this is ideal shoulder posture.

- **Thoracic spine (upper back)**

Ideal spinal position of the upper back should display a mild backwards curve. If the curve is excessive, the chest will look flat and the shoulders will be slouched forward. Focus on sticking your chest up and out to create proper alignment of the upper back. The "thumbs up and out" movement will also help set proper upper back alignment.

17

www.cpifitness.com   www.definitiveropes.com

- **Lumbar spine (lower back)**

The lower spine and hips are directly related, so aligning your lower back ensures proper alignment of your hips. The lumbar spine should have a slight inward curve. A quick and easy judge to assess lumbar spine alignment is to look at your waist band. If you waist band is level and parallel to the floor lumbar alignment should be ideal. If your waist band is tilted up, tilt your hips forward and hold this position when performing rope movements. This will help train the spine to develop strength in the correct lumbar position and should correct your posture overtime.

Knowing what proper positioning feels like makes it easier to transition that good posture to your battling rope training program. If the spine is not kept properly aligned, muscle imbalances that limit the amount of force you can produce may result. Accordingly, you should use the stabilization exercises before transitioning into power movements. Doing so will allow your body to adapt through development of good posture and core stabilization, preparing you for the more advanced and taxing power movements.

Finally, it is worthwhile to note that spinal alignment is not only important to proper battling-rope movements, it is also important to your general health and fitness. If you do not currently have proper posture, you may want to practice spinal positions in the mirror, working toward better understanding what proper positioning feels like as an additional component to both a healthy lifestyle and battling-ropes training.

Section 2: Stabilization Exercises

Figure Eights

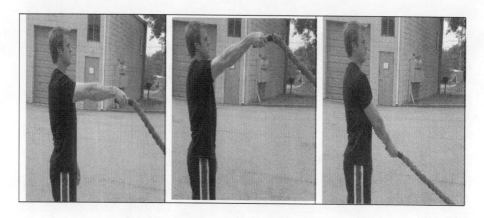

Purpose	• Improve activation and strength of the rotator cuff • Improve glenohumeral joint (shoulder) stability
Set-up	• Stand tall holding one rope • Overhand grip
Performance	• Extend arm forward holding onto rope • Trace Figure 8 pattern with arm • 10 – 15 repetitions can be performed on each arm [Is there a reason that sometimes you suggest a # of reps and sometimes you don't? Thinking should be consistent one way or the other?]
Tips	• Hold a tall posture maintaining core stability • Depress and retract shoulders to better engage shoulder stabilizers

I.Y.T.

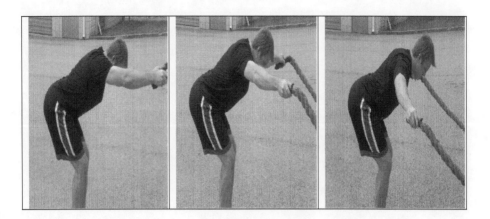

Purpose	<ul><li>Improve activation and strength of the rotator cuff</li><li>Improve glenohumeral joint (shoulder) stability</li><li>Engage lower trapezious</li></ul>
Set-up	<ul><li>Hold ropes in both hands</li><li>Use overhand grip</li><li>Lean forward till torso is near parallel to floor</li></ul>
Performance	<ul><li>Maintain neutral/straight spine</li><li>Lift arms straight above head into a "I" position</li><li>Relax arms and then extend arms 45° from head into a "Y" position</li><li>Relax arms then extend out 90° from sides into a "T" position</li><li>5 reps at each letter position for a total of 15 repetitions</li></ul>
Tips	<ul><li>Keep shoulders depressed</li><li>Work to lift arms as high as possible in each letter position</li><li>Tuck head back mimicking a double chin through movements</li></ul>

Internal/External Rotation Waves

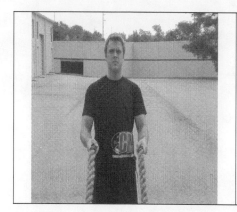 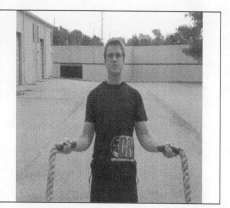

Purpose	• Improve activation and strength of the rotator cuff • Improve glenohumeral joint (shoulder) stability • Improve pectoralis strength
Set-up	• Hold both ropes with an overhand grip • Hold elbows against side of body • Bend arms 90° at elbows
Performance	• Elbows locked into sides quickly pull hands close together • Then quickly pull hands as far away as possible • Lateral waves will be made with the rope • Perform for set amount of repetitions or time
Tips	• Keeping the elbows pinned into your torso is key • Elbows drifting up cause excess strain on the shoulder joint

Core Side to Side Wave

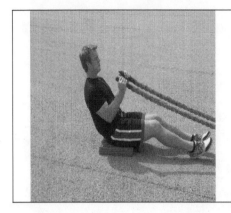
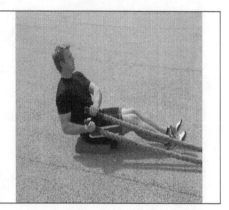

Purpose	• Improve activation and strength of abdominals • Improve glenohumeral joint (shoulder) stability • Develop dynamic stabilization of the entire core
Set-up	• Sit on floor holding ropes in an underhand grip position • Hold torso up at 45° position from floor • Feet can be flat on floor or elevated for increased difficulty
Performance	• Swing ropes from left to right side of body • No movement should come from the torso • All movement is started at the shoulders and arms • Perform for set amount of repetitions or time
Tips	• Focus on zero movement in the core • Once the 45° torso position is set, stabilization for the core muscles is engaged throughout the movement

Plank Single Arm Waves

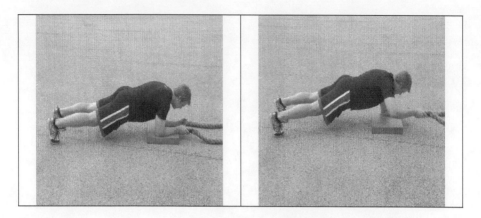

Purpose	• Improve activation and strength of the rotator cuff • Improve glenohumeral joint (shoulder) stability • Improve core stabilization
Set-up	• Start in a normal plank position • Hold one rope end with an overhead grip
Performance	• In the plank position lift one arm while holding the rope • Extended arm out and work to create lateral waves • Perform 15 reps on each arm
Tips	• Maintain a neutral spine position • Plank should be level, lifting of the hips changes the exercise

Leaning Landmines

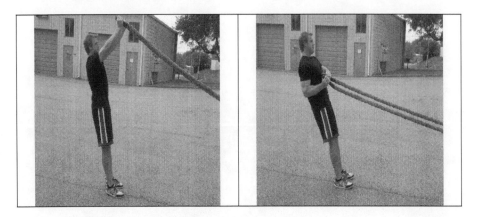

Purpose	• Improve core stabilization
Set-up	• Hold both ropes with an underhand grip • Pull ropes towards your face until they are tight • Take a slight step forward keeping tension on the ropes
Performance	• While keeping tension on the ropes, lift ropes overhead • Keeping the torso stable, lower the ropes to your left side • Return ropes overhead • Keeping the torso stable, lower the ropes to your right side • Return to center • Repeat for 10 on each side 20 reps total
Tips	• Maintain a neutral spine position • Focus on zero movement in the core • All movement should come from the shoulder joint

Wand Waves

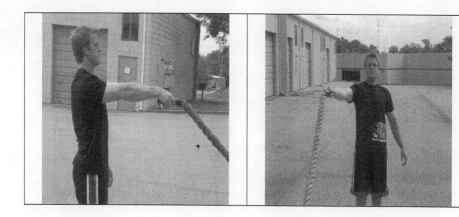

Purpose	• Improve activation and strength of the rotator cuff • Improve glenohumeral joint stability • Improve core stabilization
Set-up	• Stand tall holding one rope with an overhand grip
Performance	• Extend arm forward holding onto rope • Hold arm parallel to ground and shake arm left to right • Perform for set amount of repetitions or time • Perform for equal parameters for each arm
Tips	• Hold a tall posture maintaining core stability • Depress and retract shoulders to better engage shoulder stabilizers

Cross Body Chops

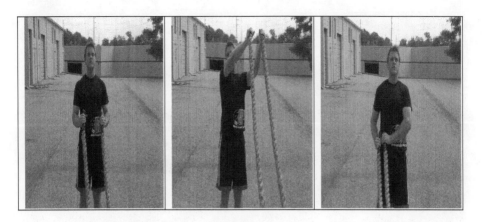

Purpose	• Improve core stabilization strength • Improve glenohumeral joint stability
Set-up	• Hold both ropes with an underhand grip • Slightly lean back keeping tension on the ropes
Performance	• Starting with ropes at left/right hip lift ropes to opposite shoulder • Quickly move ropes in a diagonal pattern across the body • Perform for set amount of repetitions or time
Tips	• Hold a tall posture maintaining core stability • Depress and retract shoulders to better engage shoulder stabilizers

Winged Vertical Internal/External Rotations

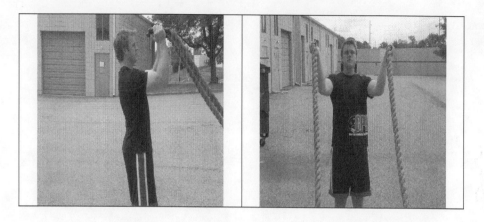

Purpose	• Improve activation and strength of the rotator cuff • Improve glenohumeral joint stability • Engage lower trapezious
Set-up	• Hold both ropes with a underhand grip • Upper arm will be parallel to floor • Elbows should be bent 90°
Performance	• Quickly move hands close together • Follow with quickly moving hands further away • Perform for set amount of repetitions or time
Tips	• Hold a tall posture maintaining core stability • Depress and retract shoulders to better engage shoulder stabilizers

Face Pulls

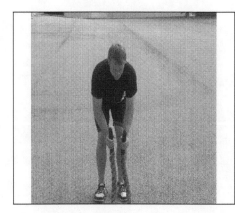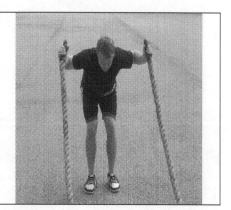

Purpose	• Improve activation and strength of the rotator cuff • Improve glenohumeral joint stability
Set-up	• Hold ropes in both hands • Use overhand grip • Lean forward till torso is near parallel to floor
Performance	• Pull ropes back and up towards face • Rotate shoulders up • Return to starting position • Perform for set amount of repetitions or time
Tips	• Depress and retract shoulders to better engage shoulder stabilizers • Keep neutral back position through movement

Plank Lean Out

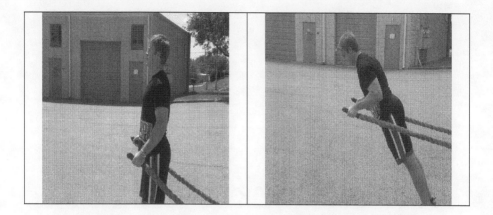

Purpose	• Improve core stabilization • Improve glenohumeral joint (shoulder) strength
Set-up	• Face away from anchor point • Hold ropes in an overhand position
Performance	• Pull ropes up towards chest to create tension • Slowly walk back keeping ropes tight • Hold neutral/straight spine for 20-30 seconds • Move torso more parallel to ground to increase difficulty
Tips	• Pull up on ropes through the entire hold • Increase duration of holds before increasing difficulty of the plank by walking back toward the anchor point

Section 3: Strength / Endurance Exercises

Bilateral Waves

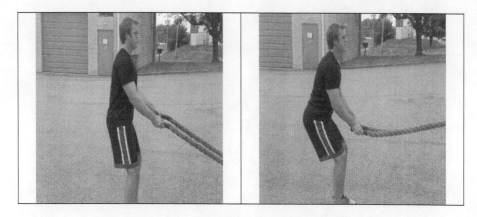

Purpose	• Improve shoulder strength • Improve core strength • Improve lat strength
Set-up	• Hold ropes in both hands • Overhand grip • Slight bend in knees with chest up
Performance	• Quickly lift ropes up until hands are chest height • Quickly pull ropes down to waist • Perform for set amount of repetitions or time
Tips	• Keep chest up and maintain a stiff core and neutral spinal position

Alternating Waves

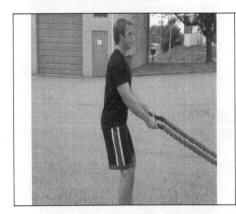 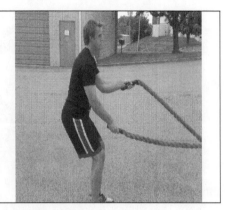

Purpose	• Improve shoulder strength • Improve core strength • Improve lat strength
Set-up	• Hold ropes in both hands • Overhand grip • Slight bend in knees with chest up
Performance	• Quickly lift one rope up until hand reaches chest height • Quickly pull rope down to waist while lifting other hand to chest height • Perform for set amount of repetitions or time at for set amount of time
Tips	• Keep chest up and maintain a stiff core to mimic an athletic stance

Punch & Pull Overhead

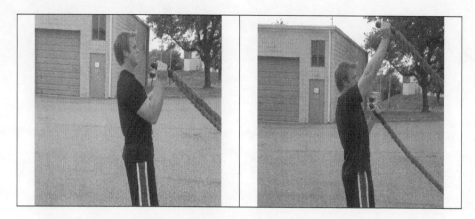

Purpose	• Improve core stabilization • Improve shoulder strength • Improve lat strength
Set-up	• Stand tall with good posture • Hold both ropes with and underhand grip • Hold ropes just below your chin
Performance	• Punch one arm into the air overhead • Simultaneously pull the rope overhead down and punch the other hand into the air overhead • Perform for set amount of repetitions or time
Tips	• Ensure you are pushing and pulling the rope with the same intensity to maintain muscular balance between muscle groups

Sprinters Underhand Grip

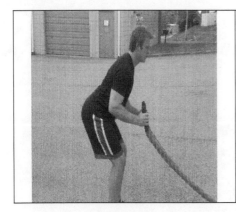 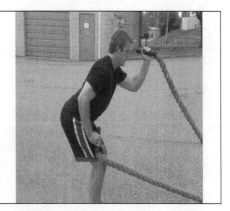

Purpose	• Improve sprinting arm mechanics • Improve lat strength • Improve shoulder strength • Improve arm strength
Set-up	• Hold ropes in both hands • Use overhand grip • Lean forward till torso is 45° to the floor
Performance	• Punch one arm up till rope end is eye level • Keep elbow bent 90° • Simultaneously pull rope at eye level down past your torso and punch opposite arm rope end up to eye level • Perform for set amount of repetitions or time
Tips	• For the upward motion, focus on punching up as hard as possible • For the downward motion, focus on punching your elbow behind you as quickly as possible

Hedge Clippers

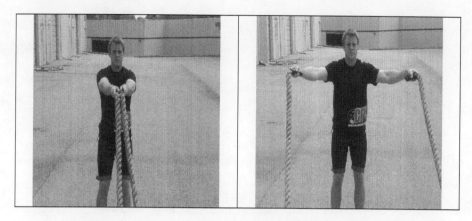

Purpose	• Improve glenohumeral (shoulder) joint stability • Improve chest strength • Improve rear deltoid strength
Set-up	• Stand tall with good posture • Hold both ropes with an overhead grip • Hold arms out straight and parallel to floor
Performance	• Starting with arms together straight in front of you • Pull arms in an arched path back until arms are straight out to your sides • Push arms back together to the start position keeping arms extended throughout • Perform for set amount of repetitions or time
Tips	• Keep arms high • Keep hips from moving back and forth by locking in your core

www.cpifitness.com   www.definitiveropes.com

Overhead Clippers

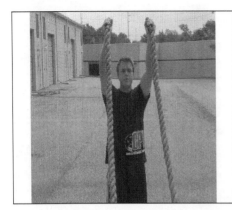 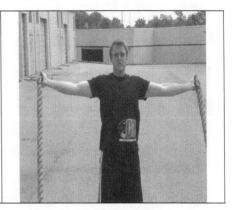

__Purpose__	• Improve core stabilization • Improve chest and shoulder strength • Improve lat strength
__Set-up__	• Hold both ropes with an underhand grip • Lift ropes directly overhead
__Performance__	• Keep arms straight and pull ropes out keeping elbows locked out • Arms will be extended straight out from sides of your torso • Quickly press ropes back overhead in an arched path • Perform for set amount of repetitions or time
__Tips__	• Keep hips from moving back and forth by locking in your core

Reverse Flies

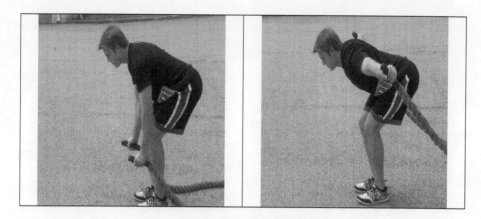

Purpose	• Improve activation and strength of the rotator cuff • Improve rear deltoid strength • Improve chest strength • Improve glenohumeral joint stability
Set-up	• Hold ropes in both hands • Use overhand grip • Stand facing away from anchor point • Lean forward till torso is near parallel to floor
Performance	• Quickly lift ropes back and out to sides of body • Then quickly pull ropes back down to starting position • Keep elbows locked out throughout movement • Perform for set amount of repetitions or time
Tips	• Focus on squeezing shoulder blades together when arms are pulled back

Swimmers Freestyle

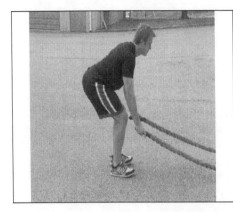 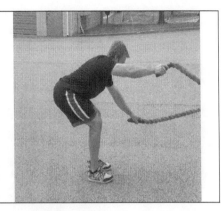

Purpose	• Improve glenohumeral (shoulder) joint stability • Engage lower trapezious • Mimic sport specific motion
Set-up	• Hold ropes in both hands • Use overhand grip • Lean forward till torso is near parallel to floor
Performance	• Lift arms until parallel to floor • Keep arms straight with elbows locked out • Simultaneously lower one arm to floor and lift one arm as high as possible • Alternate positions with arms repeated • Perform for set amount of repetitions or time
Tips	• Keep core tight • Depress and retract shoulders to better engage shoulder stabilizers

Swimmers Butterfly

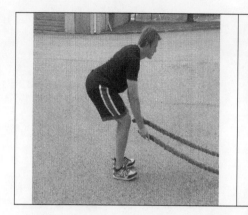 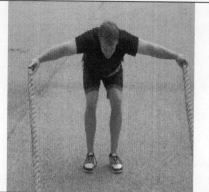

Purpose	• Improve glenohumeral (shoulder) joint stability and range of motion • Engage lower trapezious • Mimic sport specific motion
Set-up	• Hold ropes in both hands • Use overhand grip • Lean forward till torso is near parallel to floor
Performance	• Lift arms out to sides until parallel to floor • Keep arms straight with elbows locked out • Trace circles in the air mimicking the butterfly stroke • Perform for set amount of repetitions or time
Tips	• Work to increase range of motion in shoulders by making as large a circle as possible

www.cpifitness.com   www.definitiveropes.com

Stir the Pot

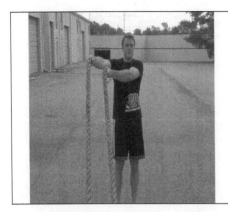 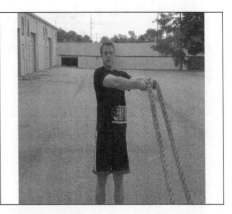

Purpose	• Improve core strength • Improve glenohumeral (shoulder) joint strength
Set-up	• Stand tall with good posture • Hold both ropes with an overhead grip • Arms will be held out straight parallel to floor
Performance	• Being the movement by shifting arms together to either the left or right side • Do not separate hands • Mimic stirring a pot with a spoon • Movement will come from the upper back and shoulders • Perform for set amount of repetitions or time
Tips	• Keep core tight • Depress and retract shoulders to better engage shoulder stabilizers • Increase size of circles/stirs to raise difficulty

Leaning Overhead Squat

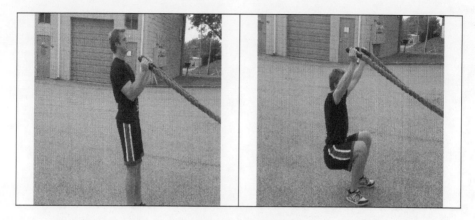

Purpose	• Improve glenohumeral joint stability and range of motion • Increase quadriceps strength • Increase glute and hamstring strength
Set-up	• Hold both ropes with an underhand grip • Pull ropes towards your face until they are tight • Take a slight step forward keeping tension on the ropes
Performance	• Lift ropes over head and pull back to keep tension on ropes • Keeping ropes overhead sit back into a squat • Once top of tights are parallel to floor return to staring position • Lower arms and repeat • Perform for 2-3 sets of 8-12 repetitions
Tips	• Depending on mobility, work to keep arms as high as possible • Tension on the ropes is crucial to safely perform this movement

www.cpifitness.com   www.definitiveropes.com

Leaning Overhead Press

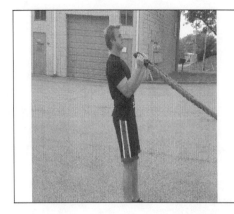 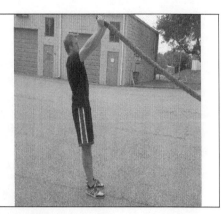

Purpose	• Improve core stabilization • Improve shoulder strength • Improve tricep strength
Set-up	• Hold both ropes with an underhand grip • Pull ropes towards your face until they are tight • Take a slight step forward keeping tension on the ropes
Performance	• Keep core tight • Gradually press ropes overhead • After arms are fully extended lower ropes back to staring position • Repeat for 2-3 sets of 8-15 repetitions
Tips	• Keep hips from moving back and forth by locking in your core • Increase difficulty by taking steps toward anchor point

Leaning Single Leg Squat

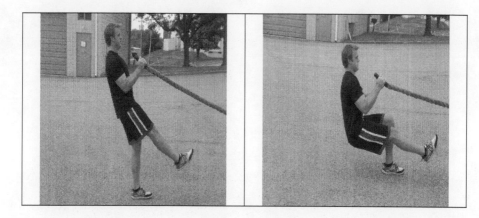

Purpose	• Improve quadriceps strength • Improve glute and hamstring strength
Set-up	• Hold both ropes with an underhand grip • Pull ropes towards your face until they are tight • Take a slight step forward keeping tension on the ropes • Lift one leg off the ground and extend leg out
Performance	• Pulling back and keeping tension on the ropes • Sit back into a squat until top of thigh is parallel to the floor • Drive heel into ground and return to starting position • Repeat for 2-3 sets of 8-12 repetitions per leg
Tips	• If quadricep strength is limited, only squat ¾ of the way down • Tension on the ropes is crucial to safely perform this movement

Single Leg RDL Wave

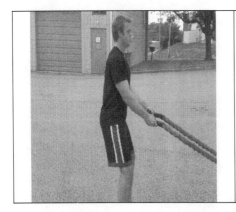 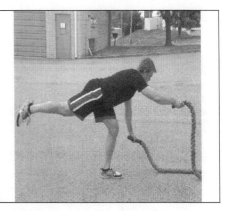

Purpose	• Improve shoulder strength • Improve lat strength • Improve glute and hamstring strength • Improve core stabilization
Set-up	• Hold ropes in both hands • Overhand grip • Slight bend in knees with chest up
Performance	• Start with alternating waves • Keeping good posture lift one leg and kick it straight back • Hinge from the hip of your planted leg • Lean forward until extended leg and torso are near parallel to floor • Repeat for 2-3 sets of 10-12 repetitions per leg
Tips	• Imagine a board being connected from your shoulder to the knee of the leg off the ground. This will keep proper spinal position • Work to feel the exercise in the glutes and hamstrings

Forward Lunge with Waves

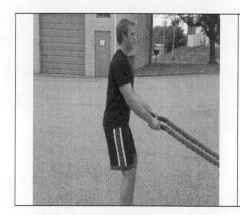 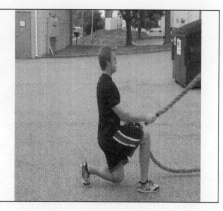

Purpose	• Improve quadriceps strength • Improve shoulder strength • Improve glute strength
Set-up	• Hold ropes in both hands • Overhand grip • Slight bend in knees with chest up
Performance	• Start with alternating waves • Take one step forward and lower your body until your knee nearly meets the floor • Keep an upright posture • Drive the lead legs heel into the ground and return to the starting position • Repeat for 2-3 sets of 10-15 repetitions
Tips	• Increase wave speed when stepping forward to keep tension on ropes • Do not relax during the lunge, keep core tight

Goblet Squat with Waves

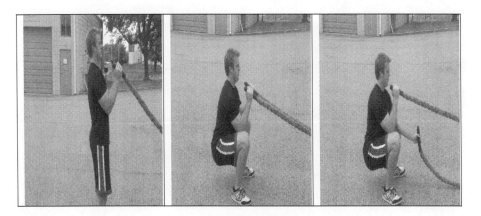

Purpose	<ul><li>Improve quadriceps strength</li><li>Improve arm strength</li><li>Improve lat strength</li><li>Improve glute and hamstring strength</li><li>Improve hip range of motion</li></ul>
Set-up	<ul><li>Hold both ropes with an underhand grip</li><li>Pull ropes toward your face until they are tight</li><li>Take a slight step forward keeping tension on the ropes</li></ul>
Performance	<ul><li>Squat down by pulling back on the ropes and "sitting back" into the squat</li><li>Descend down until elbows are resting on the inside of your thighs</li><li>Quickly extend arm out at the elbow on one arm</li><li>Simultaneously curl extended arm back in and extend other arm out</li><li>Pull both arms back with elbows at 90° and drive heels into ground to return to starting position</li><li>Repeat of 2-3 sets of 10-12 repetitions</li></ul>
Tips	<ul><li>Always keep tension on at least one rope</li><li>At the bottom of the squat push elbows into tights hard to maintain stability</li></ul>

Standing to Kneeling Waves

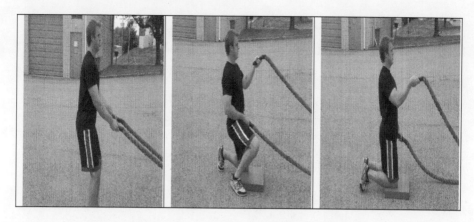

Purpose	• Improve core stabilization • Improve quadriceps strength • Improve lat and shoulder strength • Increase coordination and balance
Set-up	• Hold ropes in both hands • Overhand grip • Slight bend in knees with chest up
Performance	• Start with alternating waves • Take one step forward and lower your body until your back knee meets the floor • Pull lead leg back and rest knee on pad • Put what was your back leg forward • Drive your now forward / lead leg's heel into the ground • Return to standing position • Perform for set amount of repetitions or time
Tips	• Keep torso tight and upright throughout movement

Section 4: Power Exercises

www.cpifitness.com   www.definitiveropes.com

Power Slams

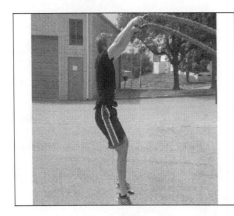 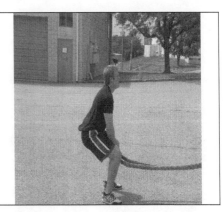

Purpose	• Improve total body power production • Improve quadricep strength • Improve glute strength • Improve lat and shoulder strength
Set-up	• Hold ropes in both hands • Overhand grip • Slight bend in knees with chest up
Performance	• Jump into the air • As you are rising lift your arms overhead as high as possible • Land with your hips back and slam the ropes into the ground • Perform for set amount of repetitions or time
Tips	• Try to slam the ropes into the ground as hard as possible

Jumping Jack Swings

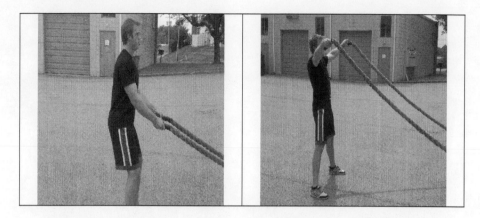

Purpose	• Improve total body power production • Improve quadricep and glute strength • Increase core stabilization
Set-up	• Hold ropes in both hands • Overhand grip • Slight bend in knees with chest up • Start with feet shoulder width apart
Performance	• Jump and shift feet out wider than shoulder width • Simultaneously lift arms up in an arching pattern until they are overhead • Jump again and shift feet back shoulder width apart and lower your arms back to starting position • Perform for set amount of repetitions or time
Tips	• When jumping and shifting feet out do not let knees cave in

Single Arm Snatch

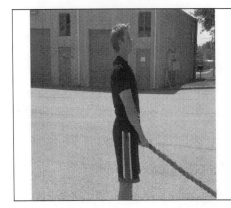 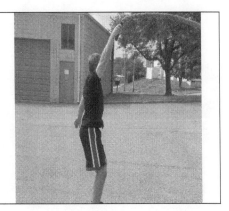

Purpose	• Improve total body power production • Improve shoulder strength
Set-up	• Hold rope in one hand • Overhand grip • Slight bend in knees with chest up
Performance	• Jump slightly and throw hips forward • Use momentum from jump to throw arm overhead • Lower arm back to starting position • Repeat for set amount of time or repetitions
Tips	• Force should be generated through hip movement • Focus on squeezing your glutes when pushing your hips through the jump

Wood Choppers

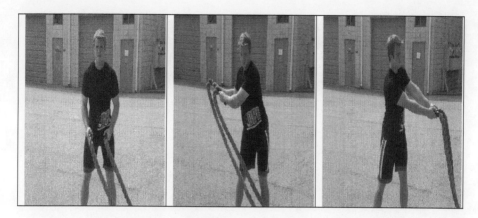

Purpose	• Improve rotational power • Improve core strength
Set-up	• Hold ropes in both hands • Overhand grip • Slight bend in knees with chest up • Stand so ropes are perpendicular to body position
Performance	• Keep feet flat on the ground • Rotate your torso with hands together to the side • Generate force from the hips and core and throw ropes to the opposite side of your body • Perform for set amount of repetitions or time
Tips	• Shoulders should rotate with the movement • When pulling the ropes back the shoulder should point directly in line with your head • Finishing position: shoulder should also be in line with head

Windmills

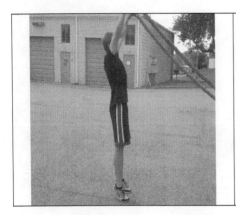 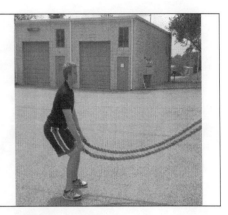

Purpose	• Improve total body power production • Improve quadricep strength • Improve glute strength • Improve shoulder strength and range of motion
Set-up	• Hold ropes in both hands • Overhand grip • Slight bend in knees with chest up
Performance	• Jump into the air • As you are rising lift your arms overhead as high • Bring ropes down quickly in an outwardly traced circular pattern • Land with your hips back and slam the ropes into the ground • Perform for set amount of repetitions or time
Tips	• Try to slam the ropes into the ground as hard as possible

www.cpifitness.com   www.definitiveropes.com

Knee Drive with Waves

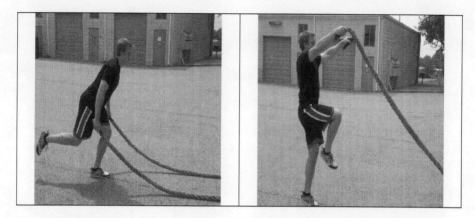

Purpose	• Improve total body power production • Improve quadricep strength • Improve glute strength
Set-up	• Hold ropes in both hands • Overhead grip • Stand on one leg • Sight bend in planted legs knee with chest up
Performance	• Jump into air off the plant leg • Lift ropes overhead • Drive the trail leg knee up into the air • Land on both feet and return to starting position • Perform for set amount of repetitions or time
Tips	• Drive knee up as fast as possible • Slam ropes into ground as hard as possible to keep up intensity

Kneeling Hop with Wave

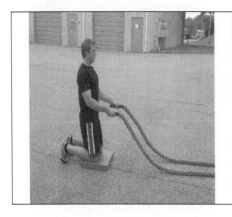 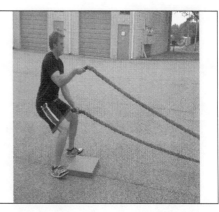

Purpose	• Improve total hip power production • Improve glute strength • Improve lat and shoulder strength
Set-up	• Hold ropes in both hands • Overhand grip • Slight bend in knees with chest up from the kneeling position
Performance	• From kneeling position rock hips back until they nearly meet your ankles • Forcible drive your hips forward • Use momentum to launch your body up into the air • Slide feet up and out and land in the standing position • Begin alternating wave pattern after landing • Repeat for 2-3 sets of 5-8 repetitions
Tips	• Keep core tight to utilize as much force generated by your glutes

Insanity (a/k/a Burpee) Slams

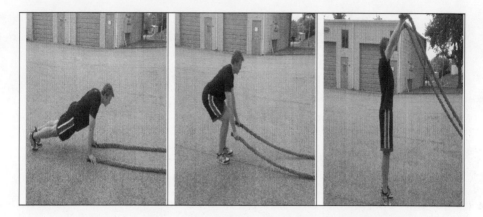

Purpose	• Improve total body power production • Improve quadricep strength • Improve glute strength • Improve lat, chest, and shoulder strength
Set-up	• Hold ropes in both hands • Overhand grip • Start in push up position with hands on ropes
Performance	• From the push up position jump and plant both feet flat on the ground towards your hands • Stand up • Jump into the air while lifting the ropes overhead • Slam ropes into the ground when landing • Jump both feet back and return to the push up position • Repeat for set amount of time or repetitions
Tips	• If completing the movement in a dynamic fashion is too difficult, eliminate all jumping from the movement and step through the positions of the burpee

Section 5: Rope Complexes

Rope complexes are the combination of multiple rope movements without rest between individual movements until the entire "complex" is complete. Complexes blend stabilization, strength, and power movements into one set that not only develops musculature but increases aerobic capacity and endurance at the same time. Repeating one movement after the next with a power emphasis elevates your heart rate and increases utilization of fat as a fuel source post-exercise. This means that after completing the complex two things have happened: (1) muscular development and (2) fat loss.

- **Muscular development**

If you lift and swing the ropes as forcefully as possible, you will stress the musculature of your entire body. This stress causes the muscles to breakdown and repair post-complex. Repaired muscles equate to more and stronger muscles. So the more complexes you do, the more muscle you create and the more force you can put into the next week's complex work. It is a positive loop: the more you put in, the more you get out.

61

www.cpifitness.com   www.definitiveropes.com

- **Fat loss**

Completing a complex with a high level of intensity taxes the aerobic system. Your heart rate and breathing rate will increase and will stay increased post-exercise. The increased heart rate post-exercise causes you to continue to use stored fat as a fuel source for up to an hour after completing the complex. Thus, because you can put this sort of intensity into a rope complex workout without a severe impact to your body's joints, complexes create the ideal result of burning fact without exposing your joints to the brute force of sprinting or running.

-- Optimal Conditions

Including timed segments for the strength and endurance movements as opposed to repetitions are the optimal means of working through any complex. Timed movements are ideal because they make it more difficult to stop and you are more likely to optimize the aerobic benefits of the complex. For that reason, having a partner who can time those segments of a complex is best.

However, if you are by yourself, you can still benefit from complexes; you simply need to commit to a specific number of repetitions for each strength and endurance movement.

Stabilization exercises will work better with a higher number of repetitions and strict adherence to perfect posture and form. For strength and endurance movements, use set amount of repetitions or intervals of 15, 20, or 30 seconds. Power movements are best performed for a set amount of repetitions because the focus is on creating as much force as you can with each movement. Five to eight repetitions will suffice. They can also be done for a set amount of time, but the intensity of each movement is the key to their effectiveness and that is better achieved through sets. Add stabilization, strength, and power in one set and you will have a tremendously effective workout that produces great results.

Complex A

	Punch & Pull	20 repetitions or 30seconds
	Power Slam	8 repetitions
	Leaning Overhead Squat	10 repetitions
	Leaning Overhead Press	10 repetitions
	Forward Lunge with Waves	20 repetitions or 30 seconds
	Freestyle Swimmers	20 repetitions or 30seconds

Complex B

	Figure Eight's	10 repetitions per arm
	Jumping Jack Swings	10 repetitions or 20 seconds
	Leaning Overhead Squat	10 repetitions
	Punch & Pull	20 repetitions or 30seconds
	Leaning Single Leg Squat	10 repetitions per leg
	Butterfly Swimmers	20 repetitions or 30seconds

Complex C

	Internal/External Rotation Waves	15 repetitions or 30seconds
	Windmills	10 repetitions or 20 seconds
	Single Leg RDL Waves	10 repetitions per leg
	Kneeling to Standing Waves	8 repetitions
	Woodchoppers	10 repetitions per side
	Leaning Landmines	10 repetitions per side

Complex D

	I.Y.T.	15 repetitions or 30seconds
	Woodchoppers	10 repetitions per side
	Goblet Squat w/ Waves	10 repetitions
	Sprinters	15 repetitions or 30seconds
	Reverse Flies	20 repetitions or 30seconds
	Core side to side	10 repetitions per side

Complex E

	Winged Internal/External Rotation Waves	15 repetitions or 30seconds
	Plank Lean out	20 second hold
	Burpee Slams	10 repetitions
	Hedge Clippers	20 repetitions or 30seconds
	Leaning Single leg squat	10 repetitions per leg
	Single Arm Snatch	8 repetitions per arm

Conclusion

Many training tools rise to popularity and some stick around for generations due to ease of use, effectiveness, and accessibility. Battling ropes meet all three of these criteria and will stay a popular choice for creating a strong and powerful body for years to come. Ropes offer years of impact-free training, and the minimized risk of injury associated can keep you training longer by avoiding injuries that sideline progress.

The gains in body-stabilization also have life-long benefits. For example, the multiple contractions of the intrinsic muscles not only develop those muscles, they also create stable and strong joints. Joints capable of supporting a load and performing powerful movements are joints that will keep you moving, functional and healthily.

Once your foundation is set with a stable body, you will be able to unleash the true training potential of the ropes to develop even more power and strength. So find a rope, anchor it to a solid surface and start swinging.   You'll be off to building muscle and

shedding fat; doesn't get any more beautiful than that.

About the Author

Brad Longazel is a leading author, strength coach, and presenter in the area of exercise science and sports performance. He is an amateur power-lifter and leads his clientele by example. He has a B.S. in Exercise Science and Sports Performance and a M.S. in Exercise Physiology from the University of Louisville. While at U of L he both lectured and assisted in course work at the undergraduate level. Brad is a certified strength and conditioning specialist through the National Strength and Conditioning Association, a certified personal trainer through the American College of Sports Medicine, and a U.S.A. Olympic weightlifting coach. He has a varied client base that includes collegiate Division I athletes, competitive powerlifters, as well as everyday athletes. His training philosophy is proper movement before pounds and to that end, he guides individuals through practical programs that produce results and help people move better. Brad has published articles on several of the most popular sites in the field of strength and conditioning. He is the co-owner of the Complete Performance Institute based in Louisville, KY.

Made in the USA
Lexington, KY
07 August 2013